I0413040

Bigger and Stronger Cookbook

One stop meal book if you are serious about it

AMARPREET SINGH

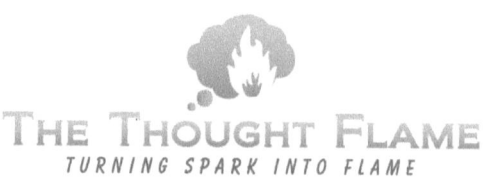

THE THOUGHT FLAME

TURNING SPARK INTO FLAME

info@thethoughtflame.com

www.thethoughtflame.com

Table of Contents

Introduction

When working on building muscle for your body, not many people understand how crucial it is to adhere to stick nutrition standards. Nutrition is everything when you are trying to build muscle and there are certain rules that you have to follow. While many people believe that "bulking up" means that they can eat whatever they want, this is not the case. Bulking up simply means eating foods that contain certain ingredients that will help your body turn those components into muscle.

There are many different things that you need in order to help your body build muscle, especially in the food that you eat on a daily basis. Some of the things you may need include:

1. Protein

Protein is an essential component to have in virtually every meal that you prepare. Protein is responsible for helping to keep your bones and muscles strong, while building new cells and tissues in the process. Your muscle tissues contain a lot of protein and the more protein you take in, the more muscle mass you will have in the long run.

2. Carbohydrates

Carbs are responsible for giving your body the energy it needs to sustain itself on a daily basis. The more you eat, the more energy you will have. If you are looking to find the energy to tackle your daily muscle building workouts, then remember to add in some carbs with every meal that you have.

3. Fats

While this may seem a little strange, another key component that you need to help you build the dream muscles that you want, you are going to have to consume some fat. Fat is responsible for helping your body to build up the insulation it needs to stay warm and to give you even more energy throughout the day.

The Most Common Myths About Building Muscle

Did you know that nine out of ten men that work out at the gym every day do not even work out correctly? You would think that with that high number most of these people would have realized it by now. Even worse then that is that also these men tend to be incorrectly as well, making their hard working efforts count for absolutely nothing. Again, these men do not even realize what mistakes they are making.

These same men also believe in many common myths regarding building muscle and I am here to tell you many of those myths are absolutely not true. Here are the top three myths that you will hear often about.

Myth #1: More Sets Equals More Muscle Growth

Most men hate long workouts. That is not a secret. They hate it so much that most men often cannot find the motivation to even do them. However, there are too many people out there that believe working out for 2 hours straight or lifting weights until they puke will help them gain more muscle mass in a shorter amount of time.

The fact of the matter is that this will not happen. When you over-train your body, you are in fact destroying the muscle mass that it already has, not adding to it. The best thing that you can do for yourself is keep your training sessions as short as possible. Around 45 to 60 minutes should suffice and it will allow your body the proper time to stimulate your muscles.

Myth #2: There Are No Exercises That Won't Help Build Muscle

This myth often makes me laugh because many people don't often realize the truth. Did you know that most of the equipment that you see in gyms today are absolutely useless? Most of the equipment that you see do not and will not help stimulate your muscles and will not help you to get ripped in the long run. It is that simple.

There are specific workouts and equipment that you should stick to if you are looking to build muscle. You want to stick to equipment that will let you freely lift a weight and you want to stick with exercises known as compound exercises such as squats and bench presses.

Myth #3: Eating Less Will Help Prevent You From Getting Fat When You Lift

When you are working out to get ripped muscles, what you eat is as important as how you workout. Many people who work out often make the mistake of working out too much and eating too little, which could cause them just to lose weight and not gain muscle, they don't eat enough protein which is important for building muscle or they simply do not portion their meal correctly at all.

The truth is that when you are working out to build muscle, you have to pay close attention to how many calories you are taking in, how much food you are eating through the day and what your meals consist of on a daily basis. You need to teach yourself how to eat properly so that you can maximize your efforts in the gym and build the muscles you have always wanted.

The bottom line here is to make sure that you eat responsibly when you are working out, do not over work yourself to gain muscle, make sure you are doing the correct exercise to maximize your workout in the gym and make sure you are preparing your meals with important components such as protein and carbohydrates. Do all of this and there is no doubt in my mind you won't get the smoking body that you have always dreamed of having.

Delicious Breakfast Recipes Designed To Help Build Muscle

Blueberry Oatmeal

Prep Time: 5 Minutes

Total Time: 5 Minutes

Makes: 1 Bowl

If you are looking for the easiest breakfast recipe to make in the morning that will help you get the muscles that you have been dreaming of, this is the recipe for you. Made with fresh fruit and egg whites, you will get the protein and healthy vitamins that you need.

Ingredients:

¾ Cup of Oatmeal, Your Choice

8 Eggs, Whites Only

¼ Cup of Water, Warm

1 Cup of Blueberries, Frozen

½ tsp of Stevia Sugar

½ Scoop of Protein Powder, Chocolate Whey

2 tsp. of Cocoa Powder, Pure

1 Tbsp. of Flaxseed Oil

Directions:

1. Mix all of your ingredients together except for the frozen blueberries. Mix these ingredients in a bowl that is microwave safe.

2. Place your ingredients into your microwave and microwave on the highest setting for 1 ½ minutes. Stir and then microwave again for 2 more minutes on the highest setting.

3. Remove from microwave and stir for at least a minute. Then add in your blueberries and

continue mixing until it is thoroughly combined with your oatmeal. Serve immediately.

Power Peanut Butter Oatmeal

Prep Time: 5 Minutes

Total Time: 7 Minutes

Makes 1 Bowl

For those who thoroughly enjoy peanut butter, this is a recipe that you are going to love. It is crafted in such a way that you will feel energized in the more while building lean muscle at the same time.

Ingredients:

1 Cup of Oatmeal, Your Favorite Brand

1 Cup of Milk, Skim

1 tsp. of Cocoa Powder, Pure

½ tsp. of Stevia Sugar

1 Tbsp. of Peanut Butter, You Favorite Brand

1 Scoop of Protein Powder, Chocolate Whey

Directions:

1. In a small microwave safe bowl mix your oatmeal, cocoa powder, sugar and milk together until all of the ingredients are combined thoroughly.

2. Place this in your microwave and microwave for 1 minute. Stir and then microwave again for another minute or until the mixture is piping hot.

3. Remove from your microwave and allow to cool for 2 to 3 minutes.

4. Last stir in your favorite brand of peanut butter and protein powder until your oatmeal is mixed thoroughly. Serve immediately.

Muscle Building French Toast

Total Time: 10 Minutes

Makes: 4 Pieces of French Toast

There is just something about French Toast that gets you going each morning. With the use of protein powder in this recipe, you can enjoy a hot and delicious breakfast meal while it helps you to pack on lean muscle.

Ingredients:

2 Eggs, Whites Only

½ Cup of Milk, Skim

2 Eggs, Large In Size

4 Slices of Bread, Whole Grain

½ tsp. of Cinnamon, Ground

2 Scoops of Protein Powder, Vanilla Whey

For Topping:

1 Banana, Whole and Mashed

1 Tbsp. of Preserves, Strawberry

1 Tbsp. of Water, Warm

Directions:

1. Mix your egg whites, milk and eggs together in a small sized mixing bowl. Next mix in your cinnamon and protein powder and beat with a whisk until everything is beaten well.

2. Take one slice of bread and dip it into your egg mixture. Let is soak for about 30 minutes or until the bread becomes soggy.

3. While your bread slices are soaking, coat a small sized pan with some cooking spray and heat on your stove over medium to high heat.

4. Place your soaked slice of bread into your pan and allow to cook for about 2 minutes on each side or until the sides turn a golden brown

color. Remove from pan and set onto a plate.

5. Using a small bowl mix up your strawberry preserves and bananas with water until thoroughly combined. Garnish your French toast with fruit mixture. Repeat process until all of your bread slices are cooked.

Pack Protein and Sweet Potato Pancakes

Prep Time: 10 Minutes

Total Time: 15 Minutes

Makes: 2 Pancakes

This recipe is perfect for those looking for a healthy and creative change to the average breakfast dish. With the use of wholesome sweet potatoes, this pancake recipe not only tastes great, but will help give you the body of your dreams.

Ingredients:

1 Sweet Potato, Medium In Size

1 Egg, Large In Size

4 Eggs, Whites Only

½ tsp. of Vanilla Extract

¼ Cup of Yogurt, Fat Free and Plain

½ Cup of Oats, Old-Fashioned

½ tsp. of Cinnamon, Ground

Directions:

1. Take your sweet potato and puncture a few holes into it using a fork. Then wrap it up in a paper towel and place into your microwave. Microwave on high for the next 5 minutes. Remove from microwave and run under cold water. Next remove the skin of the potato using a knife and set aside.

2. Using a medium sized mixing bowl, blend your oats until it reaches the consistency of a powder. Then blend up your sweet potato until it reaches a smooth consistency and mix with your powdered oats. Add in your egg whites, yogurt, eggs, vanilla and cinnamon and stir together until all of the ingredients are thoroughly combined and the batter is smooth in consistency.

3. Next coat a medium sized cooking pan with a generous amount of cooking spray and heat up over low to medium heat.

4. Then spoon about ½ cup of your batter into the hot pan and allow to cook for 2 minutes or until it reaches a golden brown color. Flip and cook for an additional 2 minutes. Remove from pan and serve on a plate. Continue cooking pancakes until all of the batter has been used up and serve immediately.

Vegetable and Bacon Omelet

Prep Time: 5 Minutes

Total Time: 16 Minutes

Makes: 1 Omelet

Omelets are the go to breakfast item for anybody who is on a diet. This recipe includes healthy and delicious turkey bacon, making this recipes savory and healthy as well.

Ingredients:

½ Cup of Mushrooms, Fresh and Sliced Thinly

5 Eggs, Whites Only

1 Egg, Large In Size

1/3 Cup of Scallions, Chopped Coarsely

3 Pieces of Asparagus, Sliced Into 2 Inch Slices

1 Tbsp. of Parmesan Cheese, Shredded and Low Fat

2 Slices of Turkey Bacon, Fresh, Cooked and Sliced Thinly

Directions:

1. Take out a large sized skillet and heat it up over medium heat. Lightly coat it with some oil of your choice and sauté your scallions, mushrooms and asparagus. Allow to sauté for about 4 minutes or until the asparagus becomes fully soft.

2. Next take out a small bowl and whisk together your egg and egg whites until thoroughly beaten. Pour over your vegetables and reduce the heat of your stove to low.

3. Allow your eggs to cook and lift the edges of the omelet to allow the uncooked egg to flow underneath the partially cooked portions. Once your egg has cooked almost completely add in your shredded cheese and turkey bacon. Let the cheese melt to your liking and then fold the

omelet on itself. Remove from heat and serve immediately.

Breakfast Style Pita Wrap

Prep Time: 5 Minutes

Total Time: 15 Minutes

Makes 1 Wrap

If you are looking for an excellent recipe that you can just take along with you on the way to work, this is certainly the recipe for you. Containing a high caloric count, you can rest assured that this wrap will help you gain the muscle that you want.

Ingredients:

3 Eggs, Whites Only

1 Egg, Large In Size

1 Tbsp. of Onion, Fresh and Chopped Coarsely

4 Mushrooms, White In Color and Sliced Thinly

1 Tbsp. of Bell Pepper, Red and Chopped Finely

3 Tbsp. of Milk, Skim

½ Of An Avocado, Sliced Thinly

1 Pita, Whole Grain, Low Fat, Halved and Slightly Toasted

½ Tomato, Small In Size, Seeded and Chopped Finely

Dash of Black Pepper For Taste

Directions:

1. Cook a medium sized skillet with a generous amount of cooking spray and sauté your bell pepper, mushrooms and onions over medium to high heat. Cook for about 4 minutes and then add in your black pepper.

2. In a small bowl mix together your milk, egg, tomato and egg white until the mixture is frothy in consistency.

3. Pour this egg mixture into your hot skillet with your vegetables and allow to cook for about 4 minutes or until the egg mixture becomes firm.

4. Remove from heat and stuff each of your pita halves with half of your cooked egg mixture. Add in your sliced avocado and take with you on the way out the door.

Classic Raisin Oatmeal

Prep Time: 4 Minutes

Total Time: 45 Minutes

Makes: 2 Bowls

With this recipe you will get the chance to enjoy delicious oatmeal that is made in the traditional way. Freshly baked, this dish will leave you feeling incredibly full while helping you to build muscle in the process.

Ingredients:

1 tsp. of Oil, Vegetable

2 Eggs, Whites Only

½ tsp. of Stevia Sugar

2 Tbsp. of Milk, Skim

1/8 tsp. of Salt

½ Cup of Oats, Quick and Cooking Variety

1 Tbsp. of Raisins

1/8 tsp. of Cinnamon, Ground

¼ tsp. of Baking Powder

½ tsp. of Brown Sugar

1 Tbsp. of Raisin, Fresh

1 Scoop of Protein Powder, Vanilla or Chocolate Whey

Directions:

1. Using a large mixing bowl, take your stevia sugar and oil and whisk together until evenly combined.

2. Then slowly add in your oats, raisins, egg whites, baking powder, protein powder, skim milk and salt. Top with your brown sugar and ground cinnamon. Cover with some plastic wrap and place into your refrigerator. Let it sit overnight.

3. The next day take out your oatmeal and place into a greased baking dish. Preheat your oven to 350 degrees and then bake your oatmeal for about 35 minutes or until the oatmeal is firm. Remove from heat and serve.

Savory Sausage and Sweet Potato Frittata

Prep Time: 5 Minutes

Total Time: 25 Minutes

Makes: 1 Frittata

This dish will leave you feeling incredibly fully and energized, especially on those days that you need it the most. The sweet potato and shredded cheese helps to bring a creative twist on a traditional dish.

Ingredients:

1 Egg, Large In Size

6 eggs, Whites Only

1 Sweet Potato, Medium In Size and Cut Into Small Sized Cubes

¼ Cup of Cheddar Cheese, Low Fat and

Shredded

1 Link Of Breakfast Sausage, Breakfast Variety and Chopped Finely

Dash of Salt and Pepper For Taste

1/8 Cup of Tomato, Seeded and Chopped Finely

1/8 Cup of Scallions, Sliced Thinly

Directions:

1. Preheat your oven to 350 degrees. While it heats up coat an small baking pan with a generous amount of cooking spray.

2. Take out a medium sized skillet and place over medium to high heat. Place your potatoes into your pan and cover. Allow to cook for 5 minutes and uncover. Add in your sausage and allow to cook for an additional 5 minutes, making sure to stir your mixture every once in a while. Cook until the potatoes are tender.

3. While your sausage mixture is cooking beat your eggs, cheese and dash of salt and pepper in a small sized mixing bowl until thoroughly beaten together. Then pour this egg mixture over your sausage mixture. Allow to cook for about 5 minutes or until the eggs turn golden brown on the bottom.

4. Transfer this mixture into your greased baking pan and place into your oven. All to back for about 5 minutes or until the top is golden brown in color. Remove from oven and top with your sliced tomato and scallions. Serve while still piping hot.

Protein Packed Banana Oatcakes

Prep Time: 5 Minutes

Total Time: 15 Minutes

Makes: 4 Oatcakes

For those looking for a healthier alternative to traditional pancakes, this is the perfect recipe for you. Simply delicious and packed full of protein, this recipe will surely not disappoint.

Ingredients:

1 Banana, Fresh and Ripe

1 Cup of Oats, Old-Fashioned

1 tsp. of Stevia Sugar

6 Eggs, Whites Only

½ tsp. of Cinnamon, Ground

1 Cup of Cottage Cheese, Low Fat

Directions:

1. Blend all of your ingredients together in a blender or a medium sized mixing bowl until the batter is at a smooth consistency.

2. Next take a skillet and spray it with a generous amount of cooking spray and heat the

skillet over low to medium heat.

3. Then spoon your thoroughly mixed batter into your hot skillet and allow to cook for about 2 minutes or until it turns golden brown in color. Flip the oatcake and allow to cook for an addition minute or until it turns golden brown in color. Slide the oatcake onto a plate to serve and continue cooking the rest of your batter.

Delicious Cinnamon and Apple Oatmeal

Prep Time: 5 Minutes

Total Time: 8 Minutes

Makes: 4 Servings

It is no secret that oatmeal is one of the easiest breakfast items to make. With this recipe you can enjoy easy to make oatmeal as well with a touch of the delicious apple flavor most people crave.

Ingredients:

1 ½ Cups of Oats, Cooking and Quick

¼ Cup of Apples, Dried and Diced Finely

4 Scoops of Protein Powder, Chocolate Whey

1/3 Cup of Dry Milk Powder, Nonfat and Optional

1 Tbsp. of Brown Sugar

¼ tsp. of Salt

1 Tbsp. of Stevia Sugar

¾ tsp. of Cinnamon, Ground

1/8 tsp. of Cloves, Ground

½ Cup of Water Per Serving Made

Directions:

1. Mix all of your ingredients together except for your water into a small sized mixing bowl.

2. To make oatmeal scoop out ½ Cup of your oatmeal mixture. Store the rest in an air-tight container. In a small saucepan mix together your oatmeal and water and heat up over medium heat. Allow to cook for about 1 minute or longer until it reaches the consistency you desire. Serve while still piping hot and enjoy.

Side Dishes, Lunch and Dinner Recipes To A Ripped Body

Mexican Style Meatloaf

Prep Time: 10 Minutes

Total Time: About 1 Hour

Makes: 8 Pieces

Meatloaf is one of the easiest dishes you can prepare for dinner. With this recipe literally all that you have to do is mixture the ingredients, bake and you are all done.

Ingredients:

1 Lb. of Lean Turkey, Ground

1 Lb. of Chicken, Ground

1 Cup of Salsa, Mild and Chunky

3 Eggs, Whites Only

¾ Cup of Breadcrumbs, Plain

1, 15 Ounce Can of Black Beans, Rinsed and Drained

1, 15 Ounce Can of Corn, Whole Kernel, Rinsed and Drained

½ of A 4 Ounce Can of Green Chilies, Fire Roasted and Diced

1 Pack of Taco Seasoning

Dash of Salt and Pepper For Taste

1, 28 Ounce Can of Enchilada Sauce, Evenly Divided

Directions:

1. Preheat your oven to 400 degrees. While it heats up take out a medium sized baking dish and coat it with a generous amount of cooking spray.

2. Then in a large sized mixing bowl, combine you chicken, turkey, green chilies, breadcrumbs, corn, egg whites, taco seasoning and black beans together until all of the ingredients are thoroughly mixed together.

3. Spoon this mixture into your baking dish and top with half of your enchilada sauce. Place into your oven and bake for the next 45 minutes.

4. Remove from your oven and top with your remaining enchilada sauce. Return to your hot oven and bake for an addition 10 to 15 minutes or until the meatloaf no longer pink on the inside. Remove from oven and serve while still hot.

Aussie Style Chicken

Prep Time: 10 Minutes

Total Time: 25 Minutes

Makes: 4 Pieces of Chicken

If you are looking for a dish that will help you change it up at the dinner table, this is the dish for you. Serve this meal with a side of healthy veggies and you will make a meal that is both satisfying and filling.

Ingredients:

2 tsp. of Salt

¼ cup of Honey

1/8 cup of Mayonnaise, Your Favorite Brand

4 Chicken Breasts, Boneless, Skinless, Rinsed, Dried and Cut Into ½ inch Thick Slices

6 Slices of Bacon, Thick Cut and Sliced In Half

¼ Cup of Mustard, Yellow

1 Tbsp. of Vegetable Oil

1 Tbsp. of Onion Flakes, Dried

1 Cup of Mushrooms, Sliced Thinly

2 Tbsp. of Parsley, Fresh and Chopped Finely

½ Cup of Monterey Jack Cheese, Reduced Fat and Shredded

Directions:

1. Once you fully prep your chicken, season it with some salt and place it into a container. Place into your fridge and leave for 30 minutes. Then preheat your oven to 350 degrees.

2. While your oven heats up, cook up your bacon in a large sized skillet over medium to high heat until the bacon is fully cooked.

3. Then using a medium sized mixing bowl mix together your mayo, mustard, onion flakes and honey until everything is well mixed.

4. Using another large sized skillet, heat up some oil over medium to high heat. Take out your chicken from the fridge and cook the

chicken in your skillet for about 5 minutes on each side or until fully browned. Transfer your fully cooked chicken to a medium sized baking dish and then top with your honey mixture. Place a generous layer of mushrooms and bacon on top and finish off with your shredded cheese.

5. Place baking dish into your oven and bake for 15 minutes or until the cheese has fully melted. Remove from oven and garnish with your fresh parsley. Serve and enjoy.

Easy To Make Chicken Salad Sandwich

Prep Time: 5 Minutes

Total Time: 10 Minutes

Makes: 2 Sandwiches

This is the perfect recipe to make if you find

yourself pressed for time and just want to enjoy something quick. Not only does it taste great, but it will help you build the muscles you have been looking to build.

Ingredients:

1 Stick of Celery, Chopped Finely

1 Tbsp. of Pine Nuts

1 Tbsp. of Onion, Chopped Finely

1 tsp. of Sour Cream, Fat Free

1 tsp. of Spicy Mustard, Brown

1 tsp. of Yogurt, Plain and Fat Free

2 Lettuce Leaves

2, 3 Ounce Cans of Chicken, Chunks, Rinsed and Fully Drained At Least Twice

4 Slices of Bread, Whole Grain

Dash of Pepper For Taste

Directions:

1. In a medium sized mixing bowl combine your sour cream, celery, mustard, pepper, pine nuts and onions together until all of the ingredients are thoroughly mixed together. Mix in your chicken gently.

2. On your slices, spread some of the mixture onto each slice. Top with your lettuce leaves and another slice of bread. Repeat and serve immediately.

Delicious Chicken Stroganoff

Prep Time: 5 Minutes

Total Time: 12 Minutes

Makes: 4 Bowls

Who doesn't enjoy a classical stroganoff dish? With this dish the chicken that you add to it packs this dish full with protein, making a dish that will help you build lean muscles in the long run.

Ingredients:

4 Chicken Breasts, Rinsed, Drained and Trimmed Of Any Fat It May Have

2 ½ Cups of Mushrooms, Fresh and Sliced Thinly

2 Tbsp. of Garlic, Minced

2 Tbsp. of Tarragon, Dried

1 Onion, Medium In Size and Chopped Finely

¾ Cup of Chicken Broth, Low Sodium

½ of An 8 Ounce Container of Sour Cream, Fat Free

Dash of Salt and Pepper For Taste

Directions:

1. Using a medium sized skillet, coat it with a generous amount of cooking spray and heat up of medium to high heat. Season your chicken breasts with your salt and pepper and place into your skillet. Cook your chicken on both sides for 2 minutes each or until each side is golden brown in color.

2. Push your cooked chicken to one side of your skillet and add in your onion to another side of the skillet. Sauté the onions until they become soft and then add in your minced garlic and mushrooms. Cook for 2 additional minutes.

3. Next add in your chicken broth and stir to thoroughly combine all of your ingredients together. Lower the heat to low or medium before adding in your sour cream. All your mixture to simmer for at least 5 minutes, making sure to stir every few minutes. Simmer until the sauce thickens. Once sauce is thickened remove from heat and enjoy.

Twice Baked Garlic Potato, Roasted Style

Prep Time: 60 Minutes

Total Time: 1 Hour and 25 Minutes

Makes: 6 Twice Baked Potatoes

This dish beautifully compliments any main dish that you make. It is savory and rich, giving you a side dish that will leave you wanting more.

Ingredients:

6 Potatoes, Medium In Size

1 Bulb of Garlic, Fresh

½ Cup of Milk, Skim

1 tsp. of Olive Oil

2 Tbsp. of Butter, Slightly Softened

½ tsp. of Salt For Taste

½ tsp. of Pepper For Taste

½ Cup of Buttermilk, Low Fat

1 ½ tsp. of Rosemary, Fresh and Minced

Dash of Paprika

Directions:

1. Place your potatoes onto a baking sheet lined with some aluminum foil and bake your potatoes for 45 to 55 minutes or until tender in a 400 degree heated oven.

2. As soon as you place your potatoes in the oven, remove the layer of skin from your bulb of garlic and cover garlic with aluminum foil. Add your garlic into your oven and allow to bake for 30 to 35 minutes or until it is soft. Remove garlic from oven and allow to cool for 10 minutes. Once potatoes are fully back allow to cool for 10 minutes as well.

3. Next cut out a thin slice off the top of each of your potatoes and scoop out the insides until you are left with a thin shell. Place the insides into a small sized mixing bowl. Add in your softened butter with your potato pulp and mash until it reaches a soft consistency.

4. Next cut the top off of your head of garlic and squeeze the garlic out into your mixing bowl of mashed potatoes. Then add in your skim milk, salt, pepper, buttermilk and rosemary. Mash together until all of the ingredients are thoroughly combined.

5. Spoon your mashed potatoes into the shells of your baked potatoes and place onto your aluminum foil lined baking sheet. Place back into your oven and bake at 425 degree for 25 minutes. Remove your twice baked potatoes from the oven and garnish with a dash of paprika. Serve immediately.

Classic Pesto Pasta With Chicken

Prep Time: About 10 Minutes

Total Time: 15 Minutes

Makes: 2 Bowls of Pasta

One of the best ways to bulk up fast is to consume lots of carbs. This dish is packed full of nutritious carbohydrates and will help get you on the road to having the body of your dreams.

Ingredients:

4 Ounces of Ziti, Whole Grain

25 Leaves of Basil, Fresh and Chopped Finely

2 Tbsp. of Parmesan Cheese, Grated

1 Tbsp. of Olive Oil, Extra Virgin

1 tsp. of Garlic, Minced

Dash of Salt and Pepper For Taste

2 Tbsp. of Pine Nuts, Crushed

1 Tbsp. of Water, Warm

1 Chicken Breast, Skinless, Boneless and Trimmed of Fat

Directions:

1. Prepare your pasta by boiling it in some water with some salt. Cook the pasta until it becomes al dente. Drain and set aside.

2. While the pasta is cooking, use a large sized mixing bowl and combine your pine nuts, basil, oil, garlic until the ingredients are mixed well. Then use a medium sized skillet, coat with some cooking spray and heat the skillet over medium to high heat.

3. Cook your chicken in your skilled and once the chicken is almost cooked fully, stir in your fresh pesto mixture, salt, pepper and grated Parmesan. Reduce the heat and cook until your

chicken is fully cooked.

4. Add to your pasta and gently toss to combine. Serve and enjoy.

Savory Chicken Cacciatore

Prep Time: 10 Minutes

Total Time: 45 Minutes

Serves: 4 Plates

This recipe is an excellent one to make if both you and your significant other are trying to gain some muscle. Great to make for lunch or dinner.

Ingredients:

1 Tbsp. of Oil, Vegetable

6 Ounces of Pasta, Quinoa Rotelle

½ Cup of Mushrooms, Fresh and Sliced Thinly

4 Chicken Breasts. Skinless, Boneless and Trimmed of Fat

1 Clove of Garlic, Minced

½ Of An Onion, Medium In Size and Chopped Finely

½ Cup of Red Wine, Dry

1 tsp. of Oregano, Dried

1, 28 Ounce Can of Tomatoes, Plum and With Juice Added

1 Bay Leaf

½ Cup of Parsley, Chopped

Directions:

1. Using a large sized skillet, place it over medium to high heat and add in your chicken with your vegetable oil. Cook chicken until it is fully browned. Then add in your garlic, garlic and mushrooms. Sauté until the onions become tender.

2. Then add in your bay leaf, tomatoes and dry wine to your vegetable mixture. Reduce the heat to low and cover. Allow to simmer for the next 30 to 35 minutes or until the chicken has been fully cooked through and the sauce reaches a thick consistency. Make sure to stir once in a while.

3. While your mixture simmers, cook your pasta in a pot with water and salt until the pasta is al dente.

4. Add in your cooked pasta with ¼ cup of the water the pasta cooked in to your chicken mixture. Allow to cook for 2 minutes, making sure to mix well so that the pasta mixes evenly. Remove your bay leaf and top with your fresh parsley. Serve immediately.

Fresh Chicken Alfredo With Some Mushrooms

Prep Time: 10 Minutes

Total Time: 25 Minutes

Makes: 1 Plate

If you are looking for the perfect dish to serve on pasta night, this is the dish for you. The shitake mushrooms help give this dish a rich flavor that will leave your mouth watering.

Ingredients:

2 Tbsp. of Olive Oil

2 Chicken Breasts, Skinless, Boneless and Trimmed of Fat

2 Ounces of Mushrooms, Shitake, Stems Chopped and Sliced thinly

3 Cloves of Garlic, Minced

2 Tbsp. of Lemon Juice

2 tsp. of Lemon Zest, Freshly Grated

½ Cup of Parmesan Cheese, Grated

½ Cup of Basil, Fresh and Chopped Finely

8 Ounces of Fettuccini, Whole Wheat

Dash of Salt and Pepper For Taste

Directions:

1. In a large pot, bring some water to a boil with some salt. Add in your pasta and allow to cook until al dente.

2. Using a large non stick skillet, heat it up over medium to high heat. Add in your finely sliced chicken and cook for the next 4 minutes or until golden brown in color. Then add in your mushrooms and garlic. Cook for an additional 5 minutes or until the mushrooms are tender.

3. Stir in your salt, lemon juice, pepper and lemon zest until thoroughly combined. Remove your mixture from heat and set aside.

4. After your pasta finishes cooking drain it, but make sure that you save ½ cup of the water that the pasta has cooked in.

5. Add in your pasta, water, fresh basil and parmesan cheese to your skillet mixture and toss gently until everything is mixed thoroughly. Serve while dish is still warm.

Filling Broccoli and Fresh Squash Stir-Fry

Prep Time: 10 Minutes

Total Time: 20 Minutes

Makes: 6 Plates

This dish is a wonderful dish to make if you are

looking for a filling side dish. The squash and broccoli balance each other out nicely without over saturating your meal with too much flavor.

Ingredients:

1 Tbsp. of Lemon Juice

2 tsp. of Honey

¼ tsp. of Ginger, Ground

1 Lb. of Squash, Butternut, Peeled, Seeded and Sliced Into ¼ Inch Slices

½ Cup of Celery, Sliced Thinly

1 Clove of Garlic, Minced

1 Cup of Broccoli, Florets and Fresh

½ Cup of Onion, Sliced Thinly

2 Tbsp. of Sunflower Kernels

Directions:

1. Using a large sized skillet, coat it with a

generous amount of cooking spray and place your skillet over medium to high heat. Add in your ginger, squash and garlic into your skillet and stir-fry your vegetables for at least 3 minutes.

2. Next add in your broccoli, onions and celery into your skillet and stir fry for an additional 4 minutes or until all of the vegetables are nice and tender.

3. While your veggies are cooking, take out a small sized bowl and combine both your honey and fresh lemon together until mixed evenly.

4. Place your fully cooked veggies into a large dish to serve and pour your honey and lemon mixture over it. Toss well to coat evenly with honey mixture and top with sunflower kernels.

Greek Style Pita Pizza

Prep Time: 5 Minutes

Total Time: 20 Minutes

Makes: 1 Pizza

Pizza is always the favorite go to food, regardless if you are on a diet or not. This recipe will give you the chance to enjoy your favorite meal while still having the chance to build the muscles that you want.

Ingredients:

1 Pita Bread, Whole Grain

1 tsp. of Vinegar, Red Wine

1 Chicken Breasts, Skinless, Boneless and Trimmed of Any Fat

½ Tbsp. of Olive Oil

¼ tsp. of Oregano, Dried

¼ tsp. of Basil, Dried

¼ Cup of Spinach, Fresh

2 Tbsp. of Olives, Thinly Sliced

½ Clove of Garlic, Minced

½ of A Tomato, Seeded and Chopped Coarsely

2 Tbsp. of Feta Cheese, Low Fat

Dash of Salt and Pepper For Taste

Directions:

1. Take out a large sized skillet and coat it with a generous amount of cooking spray. Place it over medium to high heat. Place your chicken into your skillet and cook for about 5 minutes on each side or until the chicken is golden brown in color. Once chicken is cooked remove it from heat.

2. To prepare your pizza, brush your pita with some oil and place it on a small sized baking

sheet. Place into your oven to broil for at least 2 minutes. While that is occurring use a small mixing bowl to combine your oregano, pepper, olives, garlic, salt, vinegar and basil together until all of the ingredients are mixed well together.

3. Spread this olive mixture over your broiled pita. Then chop up your chicken breast into small cubes. Top your pita with your chicken, tomato, spinach and feta. Place into your oven and broil for at least 3 minutes or until cheese is fully melted through.

Succulent Baked Salmon With Steamed Broccoli and Roasted Potatoes

Prep Time: 10 Minutes

Total Time:35 Minutes

Makes: 2 Plates

With this recipe you will be able to turn boring old fish with veggies and potatoes into a feast fit for a king or queen. This recipe contains the perfect balance of calories and fat, to make a recipe that will help you build the muscles you have always wanted.

Ingredients:

1 Pound of Salmon, Wild Caught

3 Heads of Broccoli, Fresh

4 Cups of Red Potatoes, Diced

2 Tbsp. of Sriracha

1 ½ Tbsp. of Lemon Juice, Fresh

3 Tbsp. of Olive Oil

1 Tbsp. of Oregano

2 tsp. of Salt

1 Tbsp. of Rosemary, Dried

2 tsp. of Garlic Powder

1 Tbsp. of Basil, Dried

2 tsp. of Black Pepper

2 tsp. of Red Pepper Flakes

Directions:

1. Preheat your oven to 400 degrees. While it heats up take out a cookie sheet with raised edges and grease it with 1 Tbsp. of Olive Oil. Place your salmon onto the sheet.

2. In a small sized mixing bowl, combine your salt, pepper, rosemary, oregano and basil together until thoroughly blended. Sprinkle about half of this mixture on top of your salmon.

3. Then add in some lemon pepper flakes and fresh lemon juice. Take out another mixing bowl, medium in size this time and combine

your red potatoes with your oil and garlic powder. Toss with your remaining seasoning mix until all ingredients are blended well together.

4. Place your potatoes into a greased baking dish. Place your potatoes and salmon in your oven and allow to bake for 25 minutes. After this time remove your salmon from the oven and lower the oven temperature to 375 degrees. Let your potatoes continue baking for another 5 minutes.

5. Next steam your broccoli in a small sized saucepan filled with at least 1 inch of water. Place over medium to high heat and allow to steam for 5 to 8 minutes.

6. Remove potatoes from oven and broccoli from heat and serve with fresh baked salmon. Enjoy.

Classic Chili

Prep Time: 5 Minutes

Total Time: 1 Hour and 10 Minutes

Makes: 20 Bowls

Whether you need something a tad spicy or something news, this chili recipe will help you get just that. Perfect to make on a cold afternoon or night, this recipe with satisfy every craving you have had.

Ingredients:

4 Pounds of Beef, Lean and Minced

3 Onion, Large In Size and Chopped Finely

4 Cans of Tomatoes, Fire Roasted and Chopped

8 Ounces of Mushrooms, Washed and Chopped Finely

Dash of Chili Powder For Taste

2 Tbsp. of Cheddar Cheese, Shredded

1, 15 Ounce Can of Kidney Beans, Rinsed and Drained

1 Small Can of Tomato Puree

Directions:

1. Using a small sized skillet, heat up a touch of olive oil over medium to high heat. Place your onions in the skillet and sauté for a couple of minutes or until the onions are soft and translucent. Remove from heat.

2. Add another touch of oil and place your beef into the skillet. Allow to cook until fully browned. Add your onions back into the pan and cook for 1 minute. Then add in your mushrooms, kidney beans, tomatoes, puree and chili powder.

3. Reduce your heat to a simmer and allow to cook for at least 1 to 2 hours or until the beans

are soft and tender. Remove from heat and serve immediately. Top with some shredded cheddar cheese.

Bodybuilder Chicken Curry

Prep Time: 5 Minutes

Total Time: 25 Minutes

Makes: 2 Plates

If you are a fan of chicken curry, you are certainly going to love this recipe. This dish is every bodybuilders fantasy as it is packed full of carbs and protein, helping you meat your muscle gain goals.

Ingredients:

5 Ounce of Chicken Breast, Boneless and Skinless

1 Red Pepper, Whole and Cut Into Thin Slices

2 Cups of Green Snap Beans, Raw

¼ Cup of Chicken Brother, Low Sodium

1 Cup of Yogurt, Plain and Low Fat

5 Cups of Mushroom, Sliced Finely

4 Tbsp. of Cornstarch

2 Tbsp. of Curry Powder

4 Tbsp of Olive Oil, Extra Virgin

Directions:

1. Prepare your boneless chicken breasts by cutting them into medium sized cubes. Then using a large sized non-stick skillet, heat up some olive oil over medium to high heat. Add in your chicken cubes and allow to cook until the chicken is fully browned.

2. As your chicken is browning, take out another non-stick skillet and heat up some

more olive oil over medium to high heat. Add in your beans, mushrooms and pepper. Sauté until the mushrooms and beans are soft. Remove from heat.

3. Once your chicken is fully browned, add in your chicken broth, cornstarch, yogurt and curry powder. Stir the entire mixture until everything is combined well. Stir often for the next 10 to 15 minutes until the sauce begins to thicken up nicely. Remove from heat.

4. Serve your chicken curry with an equal amount of sautéed vegetables. Enjoy.

Chicken and Salsa Pizza

Prep Time: 5 Minutes

Total Time: 20 Minutes

Makes: 1 Pizza

If you are in the mood for pizza, but don't want to stick to just traditional plain cheese pizza, this is the perfect dish for you. With this recipe you will be able to enjoy 4 protein packed slices of pizza with a creative twist thrown in.

Ingredients:

1, 12 Inch Pizza Crust, Whole Wheat and Bought From The Store

1 Onion, Small In Size

12 Ounces of Salsa, Mild and Your Favorite Brand

1 Handful of Spinach, Fresh

1.5 Ounces of Black Olives, Fresh and Chopped Finely

8 Ounces of Mexican Four Cheese Blend, Shredded

10 Ounces of Chicken, Fully Cooked and Chopped Finely

Directions:

1. Preheat your oven to 350 degrees. While your oven is heating up spread your mild salsa evenly over the entire pizza crust.

2. Then add your chopped onions, black olives and fresh spinach on top of your salsa. Last top it off with your cooked chicken and shredded cheese.

3. Place into your oven and bake for the next 12 to 15 minutes. Remove from oven and allow to cool slightly before serving.

Succulent Scallop Cerviche

Prep Time: 5 Minutes

Total Time: 4 to 8 Hours

Makes: 3 Plates

Seafood fans can officially rejoice. With this delicious scallop recipe your taste buds will be happily pleased with this high protein and low fat meal. It is very easy to make and taste absolutely delicious.

Ingredients:

1 Pound of Scallops, Small In Size Preferably

^ Limes, Fresh and Juice Only

1 Tomato, Medium In Size and Sliced Finely

½ of A Red Onion, Large In Size and Chopped Finely

2 Tbsp. of Capers, Fresh

2 Tbsp. of Olive Oil

Dash of Sea Salt and Pepper For Taste

1 Stalk of Celery, Fresh

Directions:

1. Place your scallops into a small and shallow bowl. Squeeze your fresh lime juice over the scallions. Cover them with some plastic wrap and refrigerate them for the next 4 to 8 hours.

2. After 4 to 8 hours remove your scallops and drain some of the lime juice that remains.

3. Then dice up your tomato, celery, and onions. Add this along with your caper, pepper, salt and olive oil to your scallops and place into your refrigerator. Allow to chill for another hour. Remove and serve cold.

Mediterranean Style Rice

Prep Time: 5 Minutes

Total Time: 20 Minutes

Makes: 1 Bowl

If you are tired of eating the same dishes over and over again while trying to gain muscle, this recipe will certainly help bring you out of that boring routine. It is absolutely delicious and will have you coming back for more.

Ingredients:

1 Can of Tuna, Your Favorite Brand

1/3 of A Red Onion, Chopped Finely

¾ cup of Basmati Rice, Washed and Drained

¼ Of An Avocado, Fresh and Peeled

2 Tbsp. of Lemon Juice, Fresh

Dash of Salt and Pepper For Taste

Directions:

1. In a small sized saucepan, bring together your basmati rice with ½ Cup of water over medium heat. Bring your rice to a boil and allow to boil for about 15 to 20 minutes.

2. While your rice cooks, prepare your onions and add them to the rice once it has finished cooking. Meanwhile drain the oil from your tuna and add the canned tuna to your rice.

3. Dice up your avocado and add to the rice as well. Last, squeeze your fresh lemon juice to the finished rice and season with a dash of salt and pepper and serve immediately.

Delicious Slowcooker Style Turkey Meatballs

Prep Time: 10 minutes

Total Time: 6 to 7 Hours and 10 Minutes

Makes: 8 to 9 Servings

There is no other dish that you will find that can help you build the lean muscles that you are looking for than this recipe. This dish's spicy and bold flavor, it will leave you wanting more.

Ingredients:

4 Pounds of Turkey, Lean and Ground

2 Eggs, Large In Size

2 Tbsp. of Coconut Flour, Optional

1 Onion, Medium In Size and Chopped Coarsely

2, 1 Ounce Bags of Green Peppers, Frozen and Chopped

1, 1 Ounce Bag of Cauliflower, Frozen

1 Bottle of Chili Sauce, Your Favorite Brand

1 Can of Cranberry Sauce, Jelled

½ Cup of Worcestershire Sauce

Dash of Garlic Salt For Taste

Dash of Black Pepper For Taste

Dash of Salt For Taste

Dash of Cajun Seasoning For Taste

Directions:

1. Cook your veggies in your microwave according to the directions on the bags and set aside.

2. In a medium sized mixing bowl combine your ground turkey, eggs and onions together. Add in your pepper, seasonings and Worchester sauce and using you hand combine all of the ingredients together.

3. Still using your hands roll your ground turkey mix into small size meatballs. The meatballs should be about the size of an average golf ball. Place your meatballs in your slowcooker with a layer of meatballs and then a layer of your cauliflower mix. Continue making these layers until all of your mixtures have been used. Then cover everything in your slowcooker with your bottled chili sauce.

4. Cover your slowcooker and cook the

meatballs on the highest setting for the next 6 to 7 hours. Turn off slowcooker and serve.

Savory Chicken Marsala and Zucchini Noodles

Prep Time: 10 Minutes

Total Time: 25 Minutes

Makes: 2 Plates

There is no need to make bland chicken breasts anymore with this recipe. Spice up your dinner table with this protein packed dish that will please even the pickiest of eaters.

Ingredients:

2 Chicken Breasts, Boneless and Skinless

2 tsp. of Cayenne Pepper

2 tsp. of Basil, Fresh

2 tsp. of Oregano

1 Zucchini, Large In Size, Seeded and Chopped Very Finely

3 Tbsp. of Olive Oil

½ of A Yellow Onion, Medium In Size, Diced Finely

½ Bulb of Garlic, Chopped Finely

2 Cups of Mushrooms, Fresh and Sliced Finely

2 Tbsp. of Flour, Whole Wheat

½ Cup of Wine, Marsala and Dry

1 ½ Cup of Beef Stock, Low Sodium

Directions:

1. Preheat your oven to 350 degrees. While your oven heats up take out a medium sized baking dish and line it with some aluminum foil. On the foil spread 1 Tbsp. of Olive Oil evenly all over it. Place your chicken in the baking dish

and season it with some cayenne powder, basil and oregano. Place your chicken into your oven and allow it to bake for 25 minutes.

2. As your chicken bakes, take out a medium sized saucepan and set it over medium heat. Place 2 Tbsp. of Olive Oil into the saucepan and sauté your garlic, mushrooms and onion until the mushrooms become tender. Then add in your whole wheat flour and cook for an additional minute.

3. Once the mixture thickens nicely add in your dry Marsala wine and deglaze the pan gently. Then add in your beef stock and reduce the heat to a simmer. Allow your sauce to cook until it thickens up.

4. Cut up your zucchini thinly to form noodles and place onto a plate. Remove your chicken form the oven, place on top of the noodles and top off with your marsala sauce. Serve immediately.

Turkey and Cheddar Quiche

Prep Time: 5 Minutes

Total Time: 40 Minutes

Makes: 16 Quiches

This recipe makes a quiche that you will instantly fall in love with. This quiche recipe allows you to make a dish that is packed full of the nutrients you are looking for to help fuel your muscle building efforts.

Ingredients:

12 Ounces of Turkey, Italian Seasoned Preferable and Chopped Finely

¼ Cup of Spinach, Fresh and Chopped Finely

½ Cup Onions, Chopped Finely

¼ Cup Green Bell Peppers, Chopped Finely

5 Eggs, Large In Size

1 Cup of Egg Whites

¼ Cup of Almond Milk, Unsweetened

1 Cup of Cheddar Cheese, Shredded

¼ tsp. of Black Pepper For Taste

Directions:

1. Preheat your oven to 350 degrees. While your oven heats up take out a saucepan and heat up 1 Tbsp. of Olive Oil over medium to high heat. Cook your turkey until it is fully browned. Remove from heat.

2. In a medium sized mixing bowl, beat together your eggs, pepper and milk together until everything is thoroughly combined. Then stir in your cooked turkey, vegetables and cheese and mix evenly.

3. Take out a muffin tin and line it with some parchment pepper. Then distribute about ¼ cup of your mix into each of the tins.

4. Place your muffin tin into your oven and allow to bake for 30 minutes or until it is set. Remove from heat and allow the quiches to cool for 5 minutes before you serve.

Tasty Tuna Burgers

Prep Time: 5 Minutes

Total Time: 15 Minutes

Makes: 3 Tuna Patties

While you are trying to build muscle, the goal is to stick to a health and protein packed diet. But who said burgers could not be healthy? With this recipe you will be able to make burger that are high in protein and that taste great.

Ingredients:

1 Ounce of Tuna, Fresh Preferably

½ Of An Onion, Small In Size and Chopped Finely

1 Carrot, Large In Size, Fresh and Shredded

2 Cloves of Garlic, Chopped Finely

4 Eggs, Whites Only

¼ Cup of Chives, Fresh and Chopped

¾ Cup of Breadcrumbs

Dash of Salt and Pepper For Taste

Dash of Paprika For Taste

Directions:

1. Using a large sized mixing bowl, mix all of your ingredients together until everything is combined thoroughly. Split your mixture 4 times and make 4 small sized patties using your hands.

2. In a non-stick skillet grill your patties on both sides for 10 minutes or until the patties are a light golden brown in color. Serve with fresh vegetables and enjoy.

<u>Conclusion</u>

There are many delicious recipes out there for you to try and that will help you to get the body of your dreams. Hopefully throughout this eBook you have been able to find a variety of recipes that have caught your eye and that have gotten you excited to prepare them. Remember, just because you are on a strict muscle building diet does not mean that you cannot enjoy what you get to eat from time to time.

All of the recipes that are listed in this eBook will help you begin building the muscles that you want, while helping you to take in the important ingredients that you need such as carbohydrates and protein sources.

I cannot put enough emphasis on how important it is to make sure that you consume enough protein throughout the day and make sure you are not pushing your body too much when you are working out at the gym. Remember, you want to build muscle, not lose it. Make sure that you take in as much protein as you can throughout the day and try to keep your exercise workouts down to only 45 minutes to 60 minutes in length. Do that and you should be able to getting that smoking hot body you have always dreamed of having.

About Us

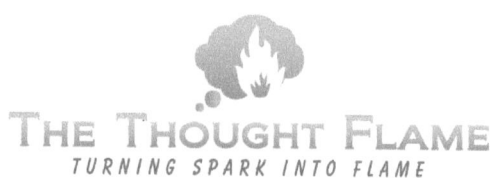

The Thought Flame is committed to add value to its customers through various books, online courses and other resources. You can learn more about us and our books at www.thethoughtflame.com.

Don't forget to check out our amazing **online video courses** at www.thethoughtflame.com/courses/ to take your knowledge to another level.

To check out our **extraordinary collection of diet/cookbooks**, visit http://www.thethoughtflame.com/category/non-fictional/cookbooks/ .

As a part of our valued relationship with our customers, we keep providing you free promotional books, courses and other stuff on subscribing with us on our site. We have a strict anti-spam policy and assure you no spam mails will be sent to your mailbox.

To subscribe with us, visit www.thethoughtflame.com.

Like our work and would like to say thanks?

Buy us a cup of coffee at www.thethoughtflame.com/coffee/

Author

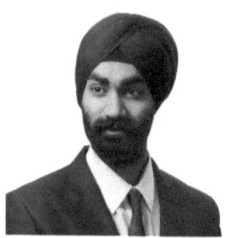

Amarpreet Singh is an avid learner and his passion for education has made him travel, work and study all across the world. He holds three masters degrees, including MBA, from top universities in Asia.

He is author of dozens of books, many of which are Amazon's bestseller, varying in various topics and categories. He also teaches many online courses having thousands of students across the world.

He has a keen interest in international affairs, economics, global poverty and politics, financial markets and entrepreneurship, and strives to be part of a community that shares the same passion.

He has worked as consultant with organizations like Airbus and The World Bank.

He loves travelling and learning about new cultures, and has been fortunate to live/work/travel/study in countries like India, China, Korea, US, South Africa, Japan, Philippines, Singapore, Canada etc., and learn about the culture and lifestyle in each of them.

To check out more of his work, visit

www.thethoughtflame.com